T3-BIE-344

*SYPHILIS is caused by a trepo-
neme known as* Treponema pallidum, *a human parasite which
ordinarily enters vulnerable surfaces of the ano-genital, oral, or
other mucous or cutaneous surfaces during sexual contact. It is
systemic from its onset, may be either acute or chronic, and is
capable of revealing itself through florid manifestations, or of
lying quiescent and unsuspected for months or even years.*

*Syphilis can imitate most of the known diseases of man, and
may involve any organ of the body at any time during its presence
in the host.*

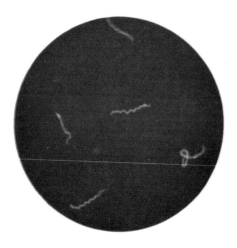

The above is one of the first color photographs of T. pallida
*exposed to serum of a syphilitic patient, then stained with fluores-
cein-tagged anti-human antibody and viewed with the aid of an
ultraviolet microscope. This is the basis for the Fluorescent Treponemal Antibody test* (FTA).

SYPHILIS

Modern Diagnosis

and

Management

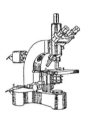

U.S. DEPARTMENT OF HEALTH, EDUCATION, AND WELFARE
Public Health Service

*The Public Health Service
gratefully acknowledges the assistance of
Dr. Sidney Olansky and Dr. Evan W. Thomas
in the preparation of this book*

Public Health Service Publication No. 743

Revised July 1961

U.S. Government Printing Office, Washington : 1961

For sale by the Superintendent of Documents
U.S. Government Printing Office, Washington 25, D.C. - Price $2 (cloth)

FOREWORD

AN eight-year decline of early syphilis ended in 1955. By 1958, early infectious cases were being reported in increasing numbers, from all areas and among all social groups.

This came as a surprise to the many persons who, for more than 10 years, had believed that "penicillin" was the magic word which would eradicate venereal disease. Belief in this myth was so strong, in fact, that it influenced an almost tragic deemphasis of the epidemiology of syphilis, from the classroom of the medical college to the office of the private physician to the department of public health.

Almost too late, we were forced by circumstances to recognize the fact that it would take more than a "miracle drug" to control this disease and keep it controlled. In the armor of penicillin itself, the chink of sensitivity began to show, and we were impelled to intensify the search for adequate alternate antibiotics.

One course of action is indicated. If we are to make real and lasting progress against this disease, we must do everything in our power now to recognize every outbreak of syphilis and to bring it under control with the greatest possible speed and efficiency.

There are no isolated cases of early syphilis. Every case of primary or secondary syphilis is related immediately to at least one additional case, and must be considered with a sense of immediacy, whether it be treated in the office of the private practitioner or in the public clinic.

Both private and public health physicians must come to recognize and discharge their individual and joint responsibilities—the private physician because circumstances are bringing an ever-increasing proportion of infected patients to his door, the public health physician because he can render the tedious and time-consuming service to epidemiology which cannot be expected of the physician in private practice. Together, these two can make an invincible team capable of the immediate and deliberate action required for the final eradication of syphilis from this country.

WILLIAM J. BROWN, M.D.
Chief, Venereal Disease Branch
Communicable Disease Center

Trade names where used are for identification only and do not represent an endorsement by the Public Health Service.

TABLE OF CONTENTS

1

Introduction

THE diagnosis and management of syphilis has become inverted over the last 15 to 20 years. Once, cases of early infectious syphilis were common. They were easy to diagnose, but their treatment was difficult. An expert was required to cope with reactions to arsenic and bismuth, and a golden-tongued orator was called for to convince patients of the necessity of completing their long-term treatment.

Today, lesion syphilis is less common. Thanks to penicillin, therapy is simple, but diagnosis has become complicated. More and more persons are receiving penicillin or other treponemicidal antibiotics for so many reasons that the signs and symptoms of early syphilis are often suppressed or modified, and the serologic reactions are atypical.

There was a period of almost two decades when, because of the difficulties of treatment and followup, syphilis case loads came to be handled principally by specialists—the bulk being diagnosed and treated in public health facilities. And this situation carried on into the period when inpatient treatment was practically eliminated, and outpatient treatment was reduced to the ultimate of simplicity.

Now, largely because of the development of penicillin therapy, but for other reasons as well, the pendulum has swung again, and the general practitioner is seeing an ever-increasing proportion of syphilitics or persons suspected of being infected. As a result, many a physician in general practice has found himself in a peculiar situation with respect to syphilis management.

If he received his formal medical training within the past 20 years, he was lucky to have been exposed to even a scant few hours of syphilology; and exceptional has been his experience if he has ever seen more than a very few "classical" cases of syphilis. On the other hand, if he was trained prior to the 1940's, chances are, his training included theoretical syphilology, and he had also the opportunity to observe many clinical cases of "classical description," the like of which he may never see again.

Unfortunately, the revolution in syphilis management occurred during the period when the fewest syphilitics were being seen by the general practitioner; and now the increasing case load is coming upon him when he has been least prepared, and is confronting him with problems which sometimes seem to call for the judgment of Solomon.

But diagnoses must be made, and the infected must be treated.

The material which follows does not pretend to be an exhaustive text on syphilology. Rather, it hopes to give in concise form and comprehensible format most of what the average physician needs to know in addition to his formal medical training to manage the average case of syphilis. But it hopes to do a little more than this.

In syphilis management, as in some other areas, the course of action often is governed by a borderline decision. Confronted with today's problems of ephemeral and atypical signs and symptoms, of weak serologic reactivity, of biological false positivity, and of increasing reactions to penicillin, the busy physician is faced by the necessity to make many such decisions.

This book also hopes to give him certain bits of practical knowledge, or rules of thumb, so that under any circumstances, he may be guided quickly to make the best of possible decisions in his diagnosis and management of syphilis.

2

The Tools of Modern Diagnosis and Management

History and Physical Examination

An accurate history is important and often essential to the diagnosis of syphilis. Such a history should include data on:

> Previous serologic tests and reason for coming to examination.
>
> Previous infection (or memory of "Bad Blood" or "Lues").
>
> Parental infection (blood tests, illness, miscarriages, still-births, etc).
>
> Treatment which might have been antisyphilitic (or patient's memory of "hip and arm" shots).
>
> Recent antibiotics (given for ailments other than syphilis).
>
> Possible exposure.
>
> Remembered signs and symptoms (lesions, bumps on genitals, rash, eye complaints, sore throat, hair loss).

In addition to the contribution of such a history to accurate diagnosis, it may prove invaluable in epidemiology.

The necessity of a careful and complete examination cannot be overstressed. Ideally, this should include a complete physical, chest fluoroscopy or X-ray, and, of course, the spinal fluid examination.

Darkfield Examination

Although syphilis is a continuum, it may be expected to pass through several rather closely definable stages—primary, secondary, latent, and late (or tertiary).

During the primary and secondary (or early lesion) stages, the *T. pallidum* may be found in the serum from the lesions or from material obtained by aspiration from regional lymph nodes, and may be demonstrated by means of a darkfield microscope. Such a demonstration, in fact, constitutes a diagnosis of primary or secondary syphilis as the case may be.

Failure to demonstrate the organism from a suspect lesion by darkfield examination may mean that:

1. The lesion is not syphilitic.
2. The patient has received antisyphilitic drugs locally or systemically.
3. Too much time has elapsed since the appearance of the lesion.
4. The lesion may be of late syphilis.

Practice is required in the proper collection of material to be examined, as well as in the identification of the organism seen. *T. pallidum* and various nonpathogenic organisms appear morphologically identical, and may be easily confused.

The lesion should be cleaned and abraded with gauze to produce superficial bleeding. The initial blood is then removed and the serum allowed to ooze from the lesion. A drop of this serum is then picked up on the surface of a glass slide and a cover slip placed over the serum. Examination under a properly adjusted darkfield microscope is then performed. If there is to be any appreciable delay in examining the specimen, the edges of the cover slip should be coated with petroleum jelly.

The expert can readily distinguish *T. pallidum* from the usual nonpathogenic spirochetes occurring in genital or skin lesions. Spirochetes from the mouth, especially around the gums, however, may be confused with *T. pallidum*.

Serologic Tests for Syphilis (STS)

Nontreponemal antigen tests. Unless specifically noted to the contrary, use of the terms "serology," "STS," "serologic test," "serologic titer," or "serologic reaction" in this book refers to nontreponemal antigen tests.

In response to invasion by the *T. pallidum,* a substance called reagin, an antibody complex, appears in the serum of the syphilitic individual, on the average, 4 to 6 weeks after infection, or 1 to 3 weeks after the appearance of the primary chancre. The presence of reagin in the patient's serum is measured by serologic tests for syphilis employing nontreponemal antigens (i.e., antigens prepared from beef heart rather than from the *T. pallidum* or certain other treponemata).

Tests commonly used to measure reagin are of two types: (a) flocculation, and (b) complement fixation. Examples of some commonly used flocculation tests are: the VDRL slide test, the Mazzini cardiolipin, the Kline cardiolipin, and the Kahn standard. The most commonly used complement fixation test is the Kolmer test.

The original Wassermann test was a complement fixation test which used as an antigen treponemes from the liver of a syphilitic stillborn. Although the Wassermann test as such no longer is performed, it is not uncommon to hear the term "Wassermann" applied to any nontreponemal serologic test for syphilis.

Although these nontreponemal antigen tests are not absolutely specific or sensitive for syphilis, their performance is quite practical, they are widely available, and their findings are, without doubt, highly indicative.

The "sensitivity" of a test refers to its ability to be reactive in the presence of syphilis, while the "specificity" of a test refers to its ability to be nonreactive in the absence of syphilis.

Some blood tests may be highly sensitive and may be particularly suited for screening, whereas others may be highly specific and more suited for use in making problem diagnoses. But the general practitioner ordinarily will need a test which combines rather high degrees of both sensitivity and specificity. And this is the kind of testing service which is provided by State, city, and other approved laboratories almost without exception.

Such tests are a definite aid in the diagnosis of syphilis in any stage, and they are used as almost the sole basis for the diagnosis of latent syphilis.

Laboratory reports based on these tests will be of two types: qualitative and quantitative. Qualitative reports will read simply:

1. **Reactive, or Positive, or 4+ (synonymous terms);**
2. **Weakly Reactive, or Weak Positive, or Doubtful, or 3+, or 2+, or 1+ (relatively synonymous terms); or**
3. **Nonreactive, or Negative (synonymous terms).**

Quantitative results are obtained by diluting or titrating the serum in geometrical progression to an end-point where it no longer is reactive. The report may be in terms of the end-point titer, or may show the degree of reaction for each titer in the serial.

An end-point titer of 1: 32 means that the serum was reactive in a dilution of 1 to 32. This may also be stated as "32 dils." Some laboratories still report quantitative Kahn or Kolmer tests by multiplying the last dilution by 4 and calling the product "Kahn units" or "Kolmer units" or simply "KU."

Most laboratories titrate to no further than an end-point of 1: 256. Above this point, reactivity has little or no additional significance. Most laboratories titrate beyond the point of 4+ reactivity, and report, for example, as follows:

1:	2	4	8	16	32	64	128	256
	4+	4+	4+	4+	4+	3+	2+	0

This type of report allows for some variation and interpretation of performance, but for practical purposes, may be considered identical to an end-point titer of 1: 32 or 32 dils.

Certain tests will not be diluted in geometric progression but rather in serial dilutions of 1: 1 2.5 5 10 25 50 100 250 500. However, their interpretation runs roughly parallel with interpretation of reactions in the standard geometrical dilution.

Quantitative serologic tests are most helpful in treatment evaluation. If the titer is established prior to treatment of a latent or late infection and followed at intervals, its descent or failure to ascend will indicate satisfactory progress. In an early case, the titer may be expected to descend if progress is satisfactory. On the other hand, if the titer rises persistently, one usually considers that the disease remains active and requires retreatment.

Ordinarily, the titer is high in secondary syphilis; but there are exceptions to this. A high titer does not necessarily mean early syphilis or even syphilis, but is strong evidence of the presence of syphilis. Some of the highest titers recorded have been in late benign visceral or cutaneous syphilis and nonsyphilitic infectious mononucleosis.

Treponemal antigen tests. Because the antigens used in the nontreponemal antigen tests are not entirely specific for syphilis, attempts have been made to prepare antigens from treponemes which would produce a specific test. Results have been rewarding; but the treponemal antigen tests up to this time have been rather difficult and costly to perform, and some have lacked the sensitivity of the nontreponemal antigen tests. They have, therefore, been considered principally as confirmatory tests in cases of doubtful diagnoses.

In 1949, Nelson and Mayer published a report on the phenomenon of Treponema Pallidum Immobilization (TPI). This employs as the antigen *T. pallida* obtained from rabbit syphilis orchitis. The treponemes are kept alive for a few hours in a special medium. When syphilitic serum and complement are added and incubated, the treponemes are immobilized; i.e., they stop moving. Present tests using this principle are considered to be specific because they employ the etiologic agent as the antigen; however, the TPI tests are less sensitive than the nontreponemal antigen tests, and become reactive later in early syphilis than nontreponemal antigen tests. *Therefore, it is possible to have a nonreactive TPI test in some cases of early syphilis.*

Other tests employing *T. pallidum* (Nichol's Strain) or extracts from this treponeme as antigen follow:

I. Whole-body antigen
    A. Viable organisms
        1. Treponema Pallidum Immobilization (1949) (TPI)
        2. Treponema Pallidum Methylene Blue (1956) (TPMB)
    B. Usually nonviable organisms
        1. Treponema Pallidum Agglutination (1953–55) (TPA)
        2. Treponema Pallidum Immune Adherence (1953) (TPIA)
        3. Whole-body Treponema Pallidum Complement Fixation (1956)
        4. Fluorescent Treponemal Antibody (1957) (FTA)
II. Fraction of organism as antigen
    A. Treponema Pallidum Complement Fixation (1955) (TPCF)
    B. Treponemal Wassermann Reaction (1957)
    C. Treponema Pallidum Cryolysis Protein (1958)

More recently antigens have been prepared from a nonpathogenic treponeme (Reiter). The one-fifth volume Kolmer complement fixation procedure using the Reiter protein fractions has shown very promising results in evaluations. This test is referred to as the Kolmer Test with Reiter Protein Antigen (KRP) or the Reiter Protein Complement Fixation test (RPCF).

The treponemal antigen tests using extracts from the Reiter treponeme (e.g., RPCF, KRP) have the advantages of lower cost and ease of performance. The nonpathogenic Reiter treponeme and the pathogenic Nichol's strain of *T. pallidum* are believed to have common protein antigen fractions. The evaluations to date of complement fixation procedures using Reiter protein antigen have shown a satisfactory degree of sensitivity and specificity. Most State health department laboratories will perform these tests on a limited basis when requested. (See Weak Reaction and Biologic False Positivity, page 47.)

Very recently a test using *T. pallida* and fluorescein-tagged antibodies has been described. It is called the Fluorescent Treponemal Antibody test (FTA). This test in evaluations has proved more sensitive than and as specific as the TPI test. It is believed that these two tests probably react to the same or similar antibodies.

The TPI test has been very helpful in the so-called "biologic false positive" problem. (See Weak Reaction and Biologic False Positivity, page 47.) However, the TPI is not a practical test, and it is very expensive. The TPCF is less expensive and can be performed in any laboratory that can perform a complement fixation test. However, it may still be too expensive for some laboratories, and there are difficulties in handling the antigen. The most recent modification of this procedure further reduces the cost, cuts the time of performance and has other advantages (tpcf–50). The Reiter protein tests can be performed very inexpensively and to date seem to be fairly adequate confirmatory tests as compared with the TPI test.

Consultation should be obtained from a syphilologist or a physician experienced in VD control when there is doubt about interpretation or correlation of a number of test results. Complete history, physical examination, date and results of serologic tests, past and present, and spinal fluid results, if indicated, should be available for such consultation.

Special purpose tests. For use in rapid screening procedures, the Rapid Plasma Reagin test (RPR) was developed. This test uses a modified VDRL antigen made more sensitive by choline chloride and tests unheated plasma instead of heated serum. The blood is collected in anticoagulant tubes (with oxalate, sequestrene, or heparin), centrifuged, and tested immediately.

This has also been adapted to perform a similar test on the plasma portion of a microhematocrit determination (Plasmacrit or PCT test). The capillary tube is nicked and divided after reading the cell volume, the plasma expressed, using a smallpox vaccine rubber bulb, and tested with RPR antigen on a slide. This has been especially useful in blood bank operation to exclude donors before collection and in screening hospital admissions, etc. Since capillary or lancet puncture blood specimen is used, this also can be useful in testing infants.

The Unheated Serum Reagin test (USR), still another screening test, is a further modification of the RPR test, but as the name implies, utilizes unheated serum instead of plasma.

Spinal Fluid Examination

Lumbar puncture in the syphilitic patient is best performed with the subject in the sitting position. This can be accomplished by having the patient straddle a straight chair, facing the chair back, and arching the spine posteriorly.

The area may be cleansed with iodine followed by alcohol or by tincture of merthiolate, tincture of zephiran, etc. A sterile spinal needle may be inserted by holding the needle only by the base. The procedure may be performed in the physician's office or the clinic without the necessity for sterile gloves and drapes.

The only means of diagnosing neurosyphilis accurately and evaluating its treatment is by spinal fluid examinations.

With the introduction of penicillin and other antibiotics, the need for spinal fluid examinations in the management of syphilitic patients is no longer quite as important as when treatment was arsenicals and bismuth. The latter therapy failed to arrest neurosyphilis satisfactorily in many cases, and it was essential to diagnose the condition because it required special therapy. Penicillin is now the treatment of choice for all types of syphilis, and it is usually capable of arresting permanently all types of neurosyphilis. Consequently, spinal fluid examinations of syphilitics are no longer as necessary as formerly.

A spinal fluid test for syphilis consists of: (1) a nontreponemal or a treponemal antigen test, (2) cell count, (3) total protein, and (4) colloidal test.

Reactive reagin tests in the spinal fluid almost always indicate past or present syphilitic infection of the central nervous system (CNS). Biologic false positive reagin tests for syphilis are rarely found in the spinal fluid. However, a reactive spinal fluid reagin or treponemal antigen test does not necessarily mean active neurosyphilis, especially in patients who have been previously treated for syphilis. Following arrest of late neurosyphilis, it may take many years for spinal fluid reagin or treponemal antigen tests to become negative or nonreactive.

Active neurosyphilis is best determined by increased cells in the spinal fluid in association with reactive spinal fluid reagin or treponemal antigen tests for syphilis. A cell count of more than 4 per cu. mm. is usually abnormal and indicative of an active infection in the central nervous system. Unless cell counts are made accurately, there is little point in doing spinal fluid examinations for syphilis. Spinal fluid containing blood or other contamination, or which is left in a warm place for 12 hours or more, will not provide an accurate cell count. Consequently, when spinal fluid is sent to a laboratory by mail or is left unexamined in a warm place for a day or more, the cell count is unreliable.

Increased total protein in association with pleocytosis and reactive spinal fluid reagin tests is also indicative of active neurosyphilis. Individuals vary considerably in their normal total protein values, but a total protein of more than 40 mgm. percent is usually abnormal. Following successful treatment, high total protein values decline slowly, and they may not become normal for a year, or even several years.

Colloidal tests of spinal fluid such as the colloidal gold test have very limited value in the management of neurosyphilis. A first zone curve indicates parenchymatous involvement of the central nervous system. However, colloidal tests are of little value in determining the activity of neurosyphilis and at times the tests yield inconsistent results, especially when made in different laboratories. Colloidal tests, like spinal fluid reagin tests, may remain abnormal for long periods after arrest or cure of neurosyphilis.

Antibiotics

Bismuth and arsenicals. Arsenicals have no place in modern syphilis therapy. There is also little, if any, indication for the use of bismuth.

Blood levels. The maintenance of a penicillin blood level ranging between 0.03 unit/ml. and 0.2 unit/ml. over a period of 10 days is adequate treatment for any stage of syphilis. This can be accomplished by a number of schedules using several penicillin preparations. Thus, the treatment can be adjusted to the schedule best suited for patient, clinic, or physician, or modified to fit public health indications.

Benzathine penicillin G. This drug is especially useful in syphilis therapy since prolonged adequate levels result from each injection (see schedules of treatment).

Procaine penicillin G with 2 percent aluminum monostearate (PAM). PAM is also a useful product since adequate levels are maintained for 3 to 4 days after an injection (see schedules of treatment).

Aqueous procaine penicillin G. This form of the drug is useful only where daily injections are indicated or desired. Since this preparation gives much higher blood levels than are needed for adequate syphilis therapy, and daily injections are necessary, there is little to recommend its use from the standpoint of the patient.

Oral medication. Oral medication is not the preferred treatment in syphilis since absorption is highly variable and patient cooperation in taking all the treatment is not always obtained.

Alternate antibiotics. When penicillin sensitivity precludes use of this drug of choice, erythromycin and tetracycline are the best alternate drugs. Recommended dosage is 20–30 gms. of erythromycin and 30–40 gms. of tetracycline given over a period of 10–15 days.

Treatment with such alternate antibiotics must be accompanied by close followup of the syphilitic patient since none of these drugs has had adequate evaluation in all stages of syphilis. Spinal fluid examinations must be done as part of followup after this type of therapy. (See Penicillin Sensitivity, page 52.)

Epidemiology of Syphilis

Treatment of a syphilitic patient, particularly in an early stage, without examining his or her contacts contributes very little to the control of syphilis.

Because persons who have syphilis usually are sexually promiscuous, and move among similar persons, and because of the characteristics of the disease itself, it is easy for syphilis to travel faster than individual cases can be sought out and treated. If treatment were confined only to obviously infected persons who volunteered for diagnosis and treatment, no measure of control ever would be effected.

In his book, "Shadow on the Land," the then Surgeon General Thomas Parran summed up the essence of syphilis control thus:

"Every early case must be located, reported, its source ascertained, and all contacts followed up to find possible infection. Enough money, drugs, and doctors must be secured to make treatment possible in all cases. Both public health agencies and private physicians throughout the country must be aligned to form a united front, and reeducated to use scientific modern methods in their joint fight against syphilis."

Every sex contact to infectious syphilis should be located, examined, and treated. Treatment may be administered on either of two bases: (1) treatment of diagnosed infected individuals, or (2) preventive or prophylactic treatment of all persons who have been exposed sexually to infectious syphilis who, although negative to present examination (physical examination and serology), may be in the incubation period or may have small undetected primary lesions.

Preventive treatment. If the patient is known to have been exposed to lesion syphilis, it is a fallacy to wait for the disease to develop to the clinical or reactive serologic stage, meanwhile allowing reinfection of treated patients and the infection of additional persons. However, every effort should be made to arrive at a diagnosis, including a complete physical examination, before administering preventive treatment.

Adequate preventive treatment may consist of 2.4 million units of either PAM or Benzathine Penicillin G.

Contact tracing. In rare circumstances, a patient with primary or secondary syphilis may have had no additional contact since the beginning of his or her incubation period; but this is most unusual. It is well to remember that two individuals naming only each other as their reciprocal contacts did not contract syphilis from each other. There must be at least one other infected individual. In addition to the source of his or her infection, the average syphilis patient may be expected to name three or four other contacts; and it is not rare for infected patients to name anywhere from 20 to 70 contacts in a 3- to 6-month period. Any one of these contacts not found and examined may develop the disease, pass it on to other persons, and become afflicted with later damaging manifestations.

Interviewing. Primary syphilis patients should be interviewed for all contacts going back 3 months prior to the onset of symptoms. Secondary syphilis patients should be interviewed going back 6 months prior to the onset of symptoms. Early latent syphilis patients should be interviewed going back at least 1 year.

Interviewing patients for contacts and tracing these contacts requires considerable time and skill, but most health departments are able and anxious to provide these epidemiologic services to private physicians—always without charge.

Public health personnel performing these services are well-trained. They are schooled in interviewing and investigating techniques which insure confidentiality and bring to treatment the maximum number of infected contacts. They can handle skillfully a great variety of personal and social problems related to sex and venereal disease.

Where such services are available, more and more private physicians are wisely taking advantage of them. Where they are not available, the physician must make every effort to do his own interviewing and to bring the contacts to examination or to report them to the health department so that they may be brought to examination.

3

The Course of Syphilis

INFECTION occurs immediately on exposure (Figure 1), but clinical and serologic evidence of syphilis is lacking for a time.

FIGURE 1

Serology of Untreated Syphilis

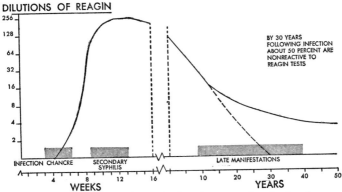

Approximately 3 weeks after infection (10 to 90 days), the chancre may appear at the site of first contact with the disease organism. Serologic tests for syphilis (STS[1]) still are nonreactive (negative), and remain so for a week or more longer before becoming reactive (positive).

About 9 weeks later (6 weeks to 6 months), secondary syphilis may appear, and ordinarily at this time, all serologic tests are reactive (positive). The lesions of primary or secondary syphilis

---

[1] In this discussion, STS refers only to tests employing nontreponemal antigens.

may disappear spontaneously, followed either by signs and symptoms of late syphilis or by a period of latency. In the later stages of syphilis, the STS are reactive. After many years, some may become nonreactive, despite possible damage such as cardiovascular or central nervous system scars, but most continue to be reactive for the life of the patient.

Treatment may change both the clinical course and serologic pattern of the disease. If the patient is treated adequately before the appearance of a chancre, it is probable that none will appear, and that his STS will remain nonreactive. If he is treated at the seronegative primary stage, his STS usually will remain nonreactive. If he is treated in the seropositive primary stage (Figure 2), his STS usually will become nonreactive within 6 months. And if he is treated during the secondary stage (Figure 3), usually his STS will become nonreactive in about 12 to 18 months. Effects of treatment after the secondary stage are variable, but as a rule, the sooner the infected patient is treated, the more marked will be his serologic response. For example, if he were treated in the early latent stage shortly after the disappearance of secondary manifestations (Figure 4), his serologic response would be similar to, though perhaps slower than, that expected following treatment of secondary syphilis.

On the other hand, if treatment be given 10 years after the onset of the disease (Figures 5 and 6), the postreatment serologic titer could be expected to change little if any. The longer the patient goes untreated, the longer will it take his STS to reach negativity after adequate treatment, if indeed it ever does. Should he have clinical lesions, they will improve with therapy though his serology remain unchanged.

Having received an optimum dosage of penicillin, it is extremely doubtful if any additional amount of antibiotics will alter the rate or nature of changes in serologic response.

FIGURE 2

Good Serologic Response to Therapy in a Typical Case of Primary Syphilis

Days after therapy	Qualitative methods [1]				Quantitative method
	VDRL slide	Mazzini	Kline	Kolmer	VDRL slide
0	W. Reactive	2	1	4	
35	Reactive	2	2	4	2 dils
80	Reactive	1	1	. . . .	
112	. . . .	. . . .	1	. . . .	
149	. . . .	. . . .	. . . . . .	. . . .	
239	. . . .	. . . .	. . . . . .	. . . .	
739	. . . .	. . . .	. . . . . .	. . . .	
1165	. . . .	. . . .	. . . . . .	. . . .	

FIGURE 3

Good Serologic Response to Therapy in a Typical Case of Secondary Syphilis

Days after therapy	Qualitative methods [1]				Quantitative method
	VDRL slide	Mazzini	Kline	Kolmer	VDRL slide
1	Reactive	4	4	4	64 dils
37	Reactive	4	4	4	32 dils
70	Reactive	4	4	4	8 dils
96	W. Reactive	3	4	4	2 dils
221	. . . .	3	2	. . . .	
306	. . . .	. . . .	. . . . . .	. . . .	
1646	. . . .	. . . .	. . . . . .	. . . .	

[1] In qualitative tests the numbers do not refer to dilutions but to the intensity of the reaction in undiluted serum.

FIGURE 4

Good Serologic Response to Therapy in a Typical Case of (Probably Very) Early Latent Syphilis

Days after therapy	Qualitative methods [1]			Quantitative method
	VDRL slide	Mazzini	Kolmer	VDRL slide
2	Reactive	4	4	32 dils
21	Reactive	4	4	16 dils
48	Reactive	4	4	8 dils
78	Reactive	2	4	4 dils
108	....	1	3	
349	....	....	....	

FIGURE 5

Satisfactory Serologic Response to Therapy in a Typical Case of Late Latent Syphilis

Days after therapy	Qualitative methods [1]				Quantitative method
	VDRL slide	Mazzini	Kline	Kolmer	VDRL slide
2	Reactive	4	2	4	8 dils
151	Reactive	4	4	4	4 dils
537	W. Reactive	4	2	4	4 dils
782	Reactive	2	2	4	8 dils
963	Reactive	4	3	3	4 dils
1078	Reactive	4	3	4	2 dils
1366	Reactive	2	2	3	1 dils
1651	Reactive	4	2	4	1 dils

[1] In qualitative tests the numbers do not refer to dilutions but to the intensity of the reaction in undiluted serum.

FIGURE 6

Satisfactory Serologic Response to Therapy in a Typical Case of Asymptomatic Neurosyphilis

Days after therapy	Qualitative methods [1]		
	VDRL slide	Mazzini	Kline
0	Reactive	3	2
294	Reactive	3	2
947	Reactive	3	2
1197	Reactive	2	3
1272	W. Reactive	2	2

[1] In qualitative tests the numbers do not refer to dilutions but to the intensity of the reaction in undiluted serum.

4

Primary Syphilis

THE first lesion of syphilis is a chancre. It is found usually in the ano-genital region, but may occur wherever the treponeme first entered the body (e.g., lip, tongue, tonsil, etc.). It is usually single, but may be multiple. It is usually an eroded hard papule, but may be quite soft. Uncomplicated, it is almost always painless. Any ano-genital lesion, however, must be suspected.

A very common site for a chancre in women is the cervix of the uterus; and such a chancre often is missed in examination of patients simply because of failure to examine the cervix.

If the primary lesion occurs at a site where regional lymph nodes are accessible, a so-called satellite bubo may often be found. This is an enlarged, discrete, rubbery, nontender node. If the primary lesion is at a site where the lymph nodes are not accessible (e.g., chancre of the anus), the satellite node could be present but not palpable.

The primary lesion will heal eventually without therapy, but the disease will continue its course.

The only absolute criterion for the diagnosis of primary syphilis is a positive darkfield examination, either from a local lesion or from a satellite bubo. However, given a healing lesion, lymphadenopathy, a rising titer, and a history of exposure, a diagnosis of primary syphilis may be made for all practical purposes.

In primary syphilis, the blood serum may be either nonreactive (seronegative primary) or reactive (seropositive primary).

Differential Diagnosis of Primary Syphilis

The following may suggest primary syphilis, but may be differentiated by the criteria indicated.

Chancroid. Lesions are usually multiple and painful. Darkfield examination is negative. *H. ducreyi* may be demonstrated from the lesion by direct stained smear examination, culture, or fluorescent antibody technique.

Granuloma inguinale. Donovan bodies may be demonstrated by direct tissue smear examination. Darkfield examination is negative.

Lymphogranuloma venereum. The early lesion is small, vesicular, and evanescent. *Treponema pallidum,* Donovan bodies, and *H. ducreyi* all absent.

Trauma. History of injury. All tests for syphilis are negative.

Herpes progenitalis. Multiple vesicles are present and usually there is a history of recurrence. All tests for syphilis are negative.

Carcinoma. Biopsy is diagnostic. Tests for syphilis are negative.

Scabies. Pruritic vesicles are present: mite is diagnostic. Tests for syphilis are negative.

Lichen planus. Lesions are pruritic. Tests for syphilis are negative.

Syphilis may be ruled out by careful history, physical and darkfield examination, and repeated STS. It is possible, however, for any disease to coexist with syphilis; e.g., a patient with syphilis may also acquire scabies, or a patient with lichen planus could also acquire syphilis, or an individual may have more than one venereal disease at a time.

Quick Reference Summary

PRIMARY SYPHILIS

Absolute diagnosis: *T. pallidum* must be demonstrated from local lesion or satellite lymph node.

Presumptive diagnosis: History of sexual exposure to a possibly infected individual within 3 months. Presence of indolent lesions, active or healing. Lymphadenopathy (possibly absent). Rapidly rising serologic titer. Nonreactive spinal fluid.

Rx: Benzathine Penicillin G—2.4 million units total (1.2 million units in each buttock) by intramuscular injection.

or: PAM—4.8 million units total usually given 2.4 million units at first session, as above, and 1.2 million units at each of two subsequent injections 3 days apart.

or: Aqueous Procaine Penicillin G—600,000 units daily for 8 days to total 4.8 million units.

or: Alternate antibiotics. (See Antibiotics, page 12.)

Prognosis: Lesions heal rapidly. Serologic titer falls rapidly to nonreactive.

Followup: Clinical inspection and quantitative STS monthly for 6 months, then at 3-month intervals for 1 year. If only one spinal fluid examination is to be done, the preferred time is 12 months' posttreatment.

Note: *Report morbidity by stage to Department of Public Health. Very important this patient be interviewed for contacts. Request epidemiologic assistance from local or State health department.*

5

Secondary Syphilis

SECONDARY syphilis is the most contagious stage of the disease. Individual patients exhibit widely varied clinical manifestations of this stage. Although constitutional symptoms such as fever and malaise are often present, the diagnosis of secondary syphilis is made primarily on the basis of lesions of the skin and mucous membranes, which may be few or many, large or small. They may be macular, papular, papulo-squamous, or pustular, but never vesicular or bullous in adults as they sometimes are in early congenital syphilis in infants. The lesions are seldom pruritic. They are bilateral and symmetrical. Moist papules (condylomata lata) frequently occur in the ano-genital region, the mouth, or other regions where moisture can accumulate between opposing skin surfaces (e.g., axillae or toewebs). The cutaneous lesions are usually dry. Frequently mucous patches of the mouth and throat are seen in secondary syphilis, as are "moth-eaten" alopecia and iritis.

As a rule, *T. pallida* may be demonstrated from any mucous or cutaneous secondary lesion, but most easily from a moist one. However, failure to demonstrate the spirochete in suspect lesions does not rule out a diagnosis of secondary syphilis.

The nontreponemal antigen tests are always reactive in this stage. Most of the treponemal antigen tests also will be reactive.

Differential Diagnosis of Secondary Syphilis

The syphilitic split papule, a condylomatous lesion occurring at the angle of the mouth, may be confused with signs of vitamin deficiency, fungus infection, trauma, or bacterial infections. However, in syphilis, concomitant lesions of secondary syphilis may usually be found elsewhere and the STS is usually reactive.

Iritis and neuroretinitis. When these are part of the secondary syphilis syndrome, they are accompanied by other recognizable lesions of secondary syphilis.

Pityriasis rosea. Pink oval papulo-squamous lesions occur along the lines of cleavage. Darkfield examination and STS are negative.

Drug eruptions. History helps. The eruption is usually pruritic and explosive. STS and darkfield examination are negative.

Psoriasis. When scales are scraped, pinpoint bleeding areas are left. There is a history of chronicity. STS and darkfield examination are negative.

Acute exanthemata. Eruption, fever, and constitutional symptoms are more pronounced and often occur in epidemics. The STS and darkfield are negative.

Lichen planus. The lesions are pruritic and violaceous. The STS and darkfield are negative.

Infectious mononucleosis. May present rash, red throat, lymphadenopathy and reactive STS (biologic false positive), but *T. pallidum* cannot be demonstrated from the skin lesion or lymph nodes. In this instance the darkfield examination is critical for diagnosis, since this disease may produce many of the signs and symptoms of secondary syphilis.

Alopecia. A moth-eaten type of alopecia is seen with secondary syphilis but is usually associated with secondary lesions elsewhere.

Any of the above conditions can occur concurrently with syphilis.

Response to syphilitic treatment is usually dramatic when the lesions are due to secondary syphilis.

Quick Reference Summary

SECONDARY SYPHILIS

Absolute diagnosis: *T. pallidum* must be demonstrated from lesion in company with characteristic skin eruptions, mucosal lesions, loss of hair, or iritis; and serology must be reactive.

Presumptive diagnosis: History of sexual exposure to a possibly infected individual within 6 months. History of possible primary lesion. History of nonreactive serology within 6 months. Suspicious characteristic lesions; any generalized non-pruritic eruptions, patchy loss of hair, iritis or neuroretinitis, mucosal lesions of mouth. High or rising serologic titer. Nonreactive spinal fluid.

Rx: Same as primary syphilis. (See Quick Reference Summary—Primary Syphilis, page 25.)

Prognosis: Lesions heal rapidly. Serologic titer reverts steadily to nonreactive, although not as rapidly as in primary syphilis.

Followup: Same as primary syphilis. (See Quick Reference Summary—Primary Syphilis, page 25.)

Note: *Report morbidity by stage to Department of Public Health. Very important this patient be interviewed for contacts. Request epidemiologic assistance.*

6

Latent Syphilis

LATENT syphilis by definition is hidden syphilis. There are no clinical manifestations of syphilis. A diagnosis usually is established on the basis of reactive serologic tests, after the possibilities of other stages of syphilis have been ruled out by physical and spinal fluid examination.

A history of exposure, or of genital lesions, or of cutaneous eruptions may be helpful to establish a diagnosis, but it is entirely possible that none of these will be remembered.

In the absence of other signs and symptoms, a reactive serologic test must be considered diagnostic of latent syphilis until the reaction is proved to be caused by something else.

No true line may be drawn between early latent syphilis and late latent syphilis. The disease is a continuum, and its progress depends very largely on the physiology of the infected individual. In the past, most authorities have defined "early latent syphilis" as syphilis of less than 4 years' duration, and "late latent syphilis" as syphilis of more than 4 years' duration, and for reporting purposes, this is preferred. Some authorities, however, classify early syphilis as infections of less than 2 years' duration. The available data suggest that the great majority of infections enter the late latent stage within 2 years after the infection, and it is probable that for epidemiologic purposes the first year is most infectious.

(See also Chapter 10—Special Problems of Modern Diagnosis and Management, page 47.)

Quick Reference Summary

LATENT SYPHILIS

Absolute diagnosis: None. (See discussion of treponemal antigen tests, page 7.)

Presumptive diagnosis: Complete absence of other signs and symptoms of syphilis. Nonreactive spinal fluid examination. No history of treatment for syphilis. Reactive serologic test for syphilis. (See also Chapter 10—Special Problems of Modern Diagnosis and Management, page 47.)

Rx: Benzathine Penicillin G—If no spinal fluid examination is done, treatment must encompass the possibility of asymptomatic neurosyphilis. In this case, 6.0 million units total, given 3.0 million units (1.5 million units in each buttock each session) at 7-day intervals.

With nonreactive spinal fluid examination, 2.4 million units given as above at a single session.

or: PAM—4.8 million units total usually given 2.4 million units at first session, and 1.2 million units at each of two subsequent injections 3 days apart.

or: Aqueous Penicillin G—4.8 million units total given 600,000 units daily for 8 days.

or: Alternate antibiotics. (See Antibiotics, page 12.)

Prognosis: Serologic titer will remain stable or decline gradually, but may remain permanently reactive.

Followup:

Early latent—Same as primary syphilis. (See Quick Reference Summary—Primary Syphilis, page 25.)

Late latent—Quantitative STS at 6-month intervals for 2 years. Either a static or a falling titer may be considered satisfactory. Persistence of reactive STS alone must *not* be considered as an indication for retreatment. (See Sero-Fastness, page 51.) At least one nonreactive spinal fluid examination, either at diagnosis or before discharge.

Note: *Report morbidity by stage to Department of Public Health.*

7

Syphilis in Pregnancy and Early Congenital Syphilis

THE signs of syphilis in the mother will depend on the longevity of the infection and the month of pregnancy. If infection and conception were concurrent or nearly so, the mother very likely would develop signs of early syphilis and the baby's chances of escaping infection are very slight. If the mother becomes infected late in pregnancy, she may not show evidence of it before she delivers, and the child may show little or no evidence of it at birth.

If the untreated syphilis in the mother is of more than 4 years' duration, the baby might escape infection.

Congenital syphilis is completely preventable or may be treated satisfactorily *in utero*. Adequate treatment of the mother during the first 18 weeks of gestation prevents infection of the baby because the *T. pallidum* probably does not cross the placental barrier until about the 19th week.

If treatment is begun after the 18th week of gestation, it amounts to treatment of the baby *in utero*. However, treatment any time during gestation is very worth while, and effects a cure of the baby almost without exception.

The cord STS. Little reliance may be placed on a cord STS. If the mother's blood is reactive, the cord blood also will be reactive. However, it is entirely possible for the mother to be infected late in pregnancy and for the cord blood to be nonreactive.

If the mother's blood is reactive, and she is treated, a reactive cord blood probably will not be indicative of congenital syphilis in the infant. Both the cord blood and, for that matter, blood from the infant shortly after birth, will contain reagin, or antibodies, causing a reactive STS. But the titer of the uninfected infant will return to nonreactive within 3 months. On the other hand, should the baby be infected shortly before birth, both the cord blood and the infant's blood may be nonreactive. The infected infant's blood will become reactive, with a rising titer, and he will develop signs of early syphilis, within 3 months after birth.

Quick Reference Summary

SYPHILIS IN PREGNANCY

Note: *Every pregnant woman should be examined for syphilis and blood tests made both early and late in pregnancy. In fact, most States require by law at least one serology during pregnancy. Inspect mother for lesions. Secondary lesions on vulva at delivery are not rare.*

Absolute diagnosis: Where clinical manifestations allow absolute diagnosis by stage, same as other syphilis.

Presumptive diagnosis: The effect of pregnancy on reagin is not clearly understood. Therefore, when there is any doubt as to previous adequate treatment, every pregnant woman with a reactive blood test, regardless of titer, should be considered to require treatment.

Rx: Dependent on stage. No additional medication is necessitated by the pregnancy.

Prognosis: Dependent on stage.

Followup: Quantitative STS in each trimester and monthly for last 3 months.

Note: *Report morbidity by stage to Department of Public Health.*

Early Congenital Syphilis

The wisest procedure when infection is suspected but unsubstantiated is to examine the mother both early and late in pregnancy, and to follow the mother serologically and both the mother and child clinically, after birth.

If there is reason to suspect that the infant might possibly be infected, it is best to check his serology monthly for 3 months.

Early congenital syphilis is similar to secondary syphilis, but often more severe in its manifestations. It may be highly infectious. It affects children under 2 years of age, and is characterized by the appearance early in neo-natal life, of some of the following:

Cutaneous or mucous membrane lesions. These are often vesicular or bullous (the exception in syphilis). The mouth, face, ano-genital, and diaper areas are most frequently involved. A positive darkfield examination of serum from a lesion establishes the diagnosis beyond a question.

Skeletal lesions. Osteochondritis of the long bones and other bone changes are common roentgenological findings. Pseudoparalysis may accompany these.

Visceral. The liver and spleen are enlarged.

Reactive STS. One should not be misled, however, by passive transfer of reagin. Periodic STS should be performed over 3 or 4 months to determine whether the titer is ascending or descending.

(See also Late Congenital Syphilis, page 37.)

Quick Reference Summary

EARLY CONGENITAL SYPHILIS

Absolute diagnosis: Darkfield positive lesions.

Presumptive diagnosis: Rising titer over 3 or 4 months. Suspect snuffles; puny, ill-nourished, wizened look. Bone lesions, particularly of long bones, are demonstrable by X-ray, but all bone lesions do not necessarily mean syphilis.

Rx: Under 2 years' duration, total dose of 100,000 units of PAM or aqueous penicillin per Kg. of body weight. PAM may be given in divided doses at 2- or 3-day intervals.

or: 50,000 units of Benzathine penicillin G per Kg. of body weight total dose administered as a single intramuscular injection.

Prognosis: Lesions heal rapidly. Serologic titer descends rapidly to nonreactive.

Followup: Same as primary syphilis. (See Quick Reference Summary—Primary Syphilis, page 25.)

Note: *Report morbidity by stage to Department of Public Health.*

8

Late Congenital Syphilis

LATE congenital syphilis is defined as congenital syphilis which has progressed beyond the second year of life. Some of the following often may be observed:

Interstitial keratitis. Most commonly appears near puberty.

Hutchinson's teeth. Widely spaced, pegged, or pumpkin-seed shaped upper central incisors with notching at the central biting edge. This phenomenon occurs in the permanent teeth only, but may be recognized in the unerupted teeth by X-ray examination.

Mulberry molars. First- or six-year molars show deficient or small cusp development with a shoulder of enamel bulging around the crown.

Eighth nerve deafness. Rare.

Neurosyphilis. Resembles that of acquired syphilis, but usually is more severe.

Gummata of the skin, bones, and viscera. Bone lesions often produce "saddle nose" or perforation of the nasal septum or the palate.

Clutton's joints. Bilateral painless effusion of the knees, often accompanies interstitial keratitis.

Quick Reference Summary

LATE CONGENITAL SYPHILIS

Absolute diagnosis: None.

Presumptive diagnosis: Reactive serology. History of syphilis in mother. Observance of stigmata characteristic of congenital syphilis. Negative history of sexual exposure. Spinal fluid may be reactive.

Rx: If spinal fluid is nonreactive, treat as late latent syphilis. (See Quick Reference Summary—Late Latent Syphilis, page 32.) If spinal fluid is reactive, treat as neurosyphilis. (See Quick Reference Summary—Asymptomatic Neurosyphilis, page 41.)

Note: *In treating late congenital syphilis in patients under 12 years of age, dosage of penicillin should be adjusted for age and weight.*

Note: *Interstitial keratitis usually will not respond to penicillin therapy alone. In addition to penicillin, corticosteroids (such as hydrocortisone) may be used locally in the eyes, usually with good response. Advice of an ophthalmologist should be sought. Administration of systemic corticosteroids has been reported to be of value in Rx of eighth nerve deafness.*

Note: *Management of late complications of congenital syphilis often requires individualized, specialized care.*

Prognosis: Serologic titer may be expected to remain the same or to descend slowly. Active lesions will heal, and further damage will not occur. In spinal fluid, cell count and total protein will return to normal, but titer may remain static or descend slowly.

Followup: If spinal fluid examination is nonreactive, quantitative serology at 6-month intervals for 2 years. If spinal was not performed initially, it should be done before patient is discharged.

If spinal fluid is reactive, quantitative serology and spinal fluid examination at 3-month intervals for first year, and at 6-month intervals for the second year. When cell count and total protein return to normal, the disease no longer is active in the spinal fluid. The spinal fluid may remain reactive for years similarly to the blood serum.

Note: *Report morbidity by stage to Department of Public Health.*

9

Late Syphilis

BEFORE considering the details of late syphilis, it is a good idea to understand the differences between early syphilis and late syphilis.

Infectiousness. Early syphilis is infectious because *T. pallida* are present in lesions. Late syphilis is not infectious, except to the fetus, and *T. pallida* cannot be demonstrated from the lesion by darkfield examination.

Destructiveness. Early syphilis lesions are acute, nondestructive, and self-healing. Late syphilis lesions are chronic and destructive.

Reinfection. Following cure of early syphilis, reinfection is common. Following adequate treatment of late syphilis, reinfection is rare.

Serology. Following adequate treatment of early syphilis, the serologic titer will become nonreactive in practically all cases. Following adequate treatment of late syphilis, the serologic titer will remain reactive indefinitely or will descend slowly over a period of years.

The classification of late syphilis includes the following:

Asymptomatic neurosyphilis
Symptomatic neurosyphilis
Cardiovascular syphilis
Late benign (cutaneous, osseous, and visceral gumma)
  syphilis

Asymptomatic Neurosyphilis

This diagnosis can be made only by spinal fluid examination. There are no clinical signs or symptoms. This is "latent" syphilis plus positive spinal fluid findings.

Examination of cerebrospinal fluid should include:

1. Cell count (lymphocytes)

    0–4—normal

    5–9—suspect

    10 or more—definitely abnormal.

2. Total proteins—normal 25–50 mgm., depending upon procedure used. (Check with laboratory on upper limit of normal.)

3. Spinal fluid test for syphilis—Kolmer or VDRL spinal fluid test usually will be reactive.

4. Colloidal tests of spinal fluid such as colloidal gold test are not specific and have very limited value in the management of neurosyphilis. (See Spinal Fluid Examination, page 10.)

The cell count and total protein are not specific tests, and pleocytosis and increased protein are common to many neurologic diseases. The spinal fluid test for syphilis is practically specific. The tests most commonly used are the Kolmer and the VDRL spinal fluid tests. The cell count and, to a lesser extent, total proteins are guides to the activity of neurosyphilis. (See Spinal Fluid Examination, page 10.)

Quick Reference Summary

ASYMPTOMATIC NEUROSYPHILIS

Absolute diagnosis: None.

Presumptive diagnosis: Reactive serology plus reactive spinal fluid, elevated cell count, or abnormal protein in the absence of other signs or symptoms of syphilis.

Rx: Benzathine Penicillin G—6.0 to 9.0 million units total, given 3.0 million units at 7-day intervals. Any benefit from more than 10 million units is doubtful and has not been demonstrated.

or: PAM—6.0 to 9.0 million units total, given 1.2 million units at 3-day intervals. Any benefit from more than 10 million units is doubtful and has not been demonstrated.

or: Aqueous Procaine Penicillin G—6.0 to 9.0 million units total, given 600,000 units daily. Any benefit from more than 10 million units is doubtful and has not been demonstrated.

Prognosis: Both blood and spinal titers will remain relatively stable or will decline slowly. Cell count will return to normal in spinal fluid within 6 months. Total protein will return to normal level in 6 months to 1 year.

Followup: Quantitative serology and spinal fluid examination at 3-month intervals for the first year, and at 6-month intervals for second year. When cell count and total protein return to normal, the disease no longer is active in the spinal fluid. The spinal fluid may remain reactive for years similarly to the blood serum.

Note: *Report morbidity by stage to Department of Public Health.*

Late Symptomatic Syphilis

The demonstrable late lesions of syphilis can be classified into
(1) diffuse granulomatous inflammations that start early in the
chronic stage, and (2) gummatous reactions that may occur at any
time during the late stage—even 30 or 40 years after infection.
The first classification includes neurosyphilis and cardiovascular
syphilis. Patients who have negative spinal fluid findings for
syphilis 2 years after infection will not subsequently develop neurosyphilis. There is no evidence from autopsies that syphilitic
aortitis starts early in the chronic stage. Both neurosyphilis and
syphilitic aortitis, as a rule, progress slowly, with the result that
physical signs of their presence may not be manifest for 8 to 15
or more years after infection.

Symptomatic Neurosyphilis

Symptomatic neurosyphilis is characterized by syphilitic damage to the central nervous system, resulting in neurologic, and often
psychotic, signs and symptoms. The blood serum is almost always
reactive, although the titer may be very low. The spinal fluid will
exhibit abnormal cell count and total protein, and will always be
reactive, excepting a few rare instances where the spinal fluid will
be normal as to cell count and total protein, and nonreactive. (So-
called burned out tabes dorsalis and occasionally in primary optic
atrophy.)

The common types of neurosyphilis are paresis, tabes dorsalis,
and meningovascular neurosyphilis. Primary optic atrophy is a
serious complication of neurosyphilis and should be checked for in
every patient.

Quick Reference Summary

SYMPTOMATIC NEUROSYPHILIS

Absolute diagnosis: None.

Presumptive diagnosis: Blood serology usually reactive, although titer may be low. Reactive spinal fluid, with elevated cell count and total protein, accompanied by neurologic and/or psychotic signs and symptoms—most commonly pupillary changes such as unequal pupils; irregular pupils; poor or no reaction to light. The more often discussed Argyll-Robertson pupil is rare compared to the above pupillary changes.

Rx: Same as asymptomatic neurosyphilis. (See Quick Reference Summary—Asymptomatic Neurosyphilis, page 41.)

Prognosis: Blood and spinal fluid titers will remain stable or descend slowly. Cell count and total protein will return to normal. Destruction will be halted. Patient may show some recovery of impaired faculties as healing takes place. Where organic damage of the nervous system has progressed to destruction of nerve cells, recovery of function will not occur.

Followup: Same as asymptomatic neurosyphilis. (See Quick Reference Summary—Asymptomatic Neurosyphilis, page 41.)

Note: *Report morbidity by stage to Department of Public Health.*

Cardiovascular Syphilis

Cardiovascular syphilis is difficult to diagnose. This is especially true in making differential diagnoses in persons more than 50 years of age. The blood serology usually is reactive, but the titer may be low; and at times the serum may be nonreactive. The spinal fluid is normal and nonreactive unless there is coexistent neurosyphilis. A history of syphilis helps in making the diagnosis. Two presumptive findings are aortic insufficiency and roentgenological evidence of an aneurysm of the thoracic aorta.

Late Benign (Cutaneous, Osseous, and Visceral Gumma) Syphilis

Gummata are sensitivity reactions to the treponeme. They may occur anywhere, excepting possibly the intestines and ovaries, but are found commonly in the skin, bones, liver, or stomach. Gummatous reactions of the skin may be solitary gummas (ulcers) or nodular-ulcerative syphilides. A biopsy may show granulomatous change and assist in making a diagnosis. Blood serology usually is reactive, often with high titer. A history of syphilis plus characteristic lesions would indicate treatment. Some confirmation of diagnosis may be made on the basis of dramatic healing of visible gummas following treatment.

Quick Reference Summary

CARDIOVASCULAR SYPHILIS AND LATE BENIGN SYPHILIS

Absolute diagnosis: None.

Presumptive diagnosis:

Cardiovascular Syphilis—Aortic insufficiency and/or aneurysm of thoracic aorta accompanied by a history of syphilis and/or a reactive serology.

Late Benign Syphilis—Suspicious cutaneous and/or osseous lesions accompanied by a reactive serology probably of high titer. Probably a history of syphilis. (Although visceral lesions may be suspected, diagnosis may depend upon therapeutic tests.)

Rx: Same as asymptomatic neurosyphilis. (See Quick Reference Summary—Asymptomatic Neurosyphilis, page 41.)

Note: *The administration of penicillin to a person with decompensation due to cardiovascular syphilis is not an emergency, and the demand is to treat the heart first and the syphilis second. The decompensated patient should be given cardiotonic drugs and diuretics first; then, penicillin may be started in full doses without preliminary heavy metal treatment. If the patient is well compensated, penicillin treatment may be begun immediately since there appears to be no demonstrable risk from penicillin alone in these cases.*

Prognosis: Late benign lesions heal dramatically. In cardiovascular syphilis, damaged or scarred vessels and valves will not be restored to normal function.

Followup: Same as late latent syphilis. (See Quick Reference Summary—Late Latent Syphilis, page 32.)

Note: *Report morbidity by stage to Department of Public Health.*

10

Special Problems of Modern Diagnosis and Management

Weak Reaction and Biologic False Positivity

Confronted by a reactive serology in the complete absence of other signs and symptoms of syphilis, the physician must decide whether or not the patient needs treatment for syphilis. Since the development of penicillin therapy, this question is not quite as critical as it once was, when therapy not only was almost untenably time consuming, but could be as dangerous as the disease itself. When there is some question as to the patient's need for syphilotherapy today, or when it is doubtful that the patient can be followed long enough to rule out biological false positivity, a course of penicillin treatment may be administered with little or no danger to the patient and with the knowledge that if he did need treatment, his syphilis will be arrested.

Nevertheless, many physicians, for many reasons, hesitate to begin syphilotherapy unless an untreated or inadequately treated syphilitic infection has been established beyond a reasonable doubt. This is becoming increasingly difficult, however, because:

a. Widespread use of antibiotics has altered serologic patterns in many cases without effecting complete cures, and

b. The prevalence of biologic false positivity (BFP), if it remains stable in the population, must constitute a higher and higher percentage of all reactive serologies as the prevalence of syphilis decreases.

Biologic false positive reactions may be either "acute" or "chronic."

The acute BFP reaction may be defined as a reactive serology in the absence of syphilitic infection, which is caused by acute illness or other stress, such as immunization. This reaction disappears in time, usually within days or weeks, without the administration of syphilotherapy. The problem is complicated by the fact that many illnesses which might produce acute BFP reactions are now treated with penicillin or broad spectrum antibiotics which, incidentally, also kill treponemes.

Many viral and bacterial infections may cause acute BFP reactions. An example is infectious mononucleosis. This disease may produce many of the signs and symptoms of secondary syphilis (see Secondary Syphilis—Differential Diagnosis, page 27), in the total absence of *T. pallida*. Whereas most acute BFP reactions are weak or have low titers, infectious mononucleosis has been known to cause extremely high titers.

Chronic BFP, a term coined by the late Dr. J. E. Moore, may be defined as a reactive serology not caused by either syphilis or acute illness, which persists for months or even years. Leprosy, collagen disease such as lupus erythematosis, and malaria may cause chronic BFP reactions. In some cases, no known cause can be found for the chronic BFP. After observing many persons with BFP reactions for years, Dr. Moore and others felt that such reactions might be significant presymptomatic indications of collagen disease.

A further serious complication in the identification of BFP reactions is that all laboratories do not perform the same serologic tests for syphilis; and those which they do perform in common vary slightly in sensitivity among laboratories, and even from time to time in the same laboratory. Therefore, it is entirely possible to have a reactive serology of low titer in one laboratory and a nonreactive in another on a split sample of blood, depending on which test was used, what antigen was employed, and who read the results. It should be added that such variations are the exception, since the performance of the approved serologic laboratory is one of the most consistent and standardized in the whole field of diagnostic medical tests.

The newer treponemal antigen tests for syphilis have been helpful in ruling out BFP reactions; but, unfortunately, they have limitations. If they are reactive, they usually indicate that the patient in question either *has* or *had* syphilis, but not that he needs treatment or has been adequately treated. (See Relapse and Reinfection—When To Re-Treat, following.)

On the other hand, a nonreactive TPI test has been considered the *sine qua non* for determining that a suspect reaction is really a BFP. But, there is no one TPI test. Very few laboratories perform it exactly alike.

It is entirely possible for a split blood sample to be TPI reactive in one laboratory and TPI nonreactive in another on the basis of sensitivity and procedure alone.

One more warning may be in order. If the patient should demonstrate a positive L.E. (Lupus erythematosis) cell preparation, a reactive serology often is considered automatically to be false. This can be misleading. Syphilis and lupus erythematosis can exist, and have been found to exist, concomitantly. By the same token, all reactive serologies in people with collagen disease are not necessarily false.

In spite of all the weaknesses, nonreactive TPI test results to date are generally the most reliable indicators of BFP reactions.

TPI's are, however, difficult and expensive to perform. The Reiter protein antigen tests, which can be performed routinely in State laboratories, may offer some solution. There is strong evidence at least that a reactive VDRL test and a reactive Reiter protein antigen test together indicate syphilis—treated or untreated.

Where available, the Fluorescent Treponemal Antibody test may be helpful. It is believed that both the FTA and TPI tests identify the same or similar antibodies. The FTA test has proved more sensitive than the TPI test as usually performed.

If one or more treponemal antibody tests cannot be obtained, and the physician cannot feel certain that repeatedly positive non-treponemal antigen tests are BFP, the wisest course of action is to treat.

Relapse and Reinfection—When To Re-Treat

Any treated syphilitic may, at a later date, need additional treatment. There are four conditions under which this is indicated. These are: (1) syphilis in pregnancy when adequacy of previous therapy is not determinable; (2) persistently active neurosyphilis; (3) relapse; and (4) reinfection. Attention should be called to one condition in which retreatment is not indicated. This is in sero-fastness, or Wassermann fastness, where no other indication for retreatment is present in addition to a reactive serology.

Syphilis in pregnancy. In pregnancy, when there is any possible doubt as to the mother's having been adequately treated, or any suspicion of an active infection, a course of therapy should be administered for the prevention of congenital syphilis. The amount of penicillin with which the mother is treated should be governed by her diagnosis.

Neurosyphilis. In neurosyphilis, if the cell count does not return to normal within 1 year, or if there is an increase in cells or protein during the followup period, retreatment is indicated. As a rule, the amount of penicillin for retreatment need not exceed 10 million units.

Relapse or reinfection? It is often difficult to determine in a given case whether one is confronted by a relapse or a reinfection. The principal significance of such a decision lies in the fact that a reinfection is treated exactly as a new case, whereas a relapse may require increased antibiotic therapy on retreatment if a low dosage schedule was used initially.

In early syphilis, the titer descends rapidly and regularly after treatment, if therapy has been adequate. Failure of this may herald either a relapse or reinfection.

A reinfection often is indicated by a new primary lesion at a site different from the last primary lesion, serology suggestive of a first infection, and history of exposure.

Because of previous sensitization to the *T. pallidum,* reinfections may produce skin and mucous membrane lesions approaching, morphologically and histologically, those of the manifestations of late benign syphilis, suggesting late relapse rather than reinfection. However, the ease of darkfield demonstration of *T. pallida* plus history should be sufficient to establish reinfection.

Relapse or sero-fastness? If syphilis remains untreated for a number of years, the serologic titer often becomes fixed. No amount of treatment will alter this appreciably. This does not mean that the patient needs retreatment. Retreatment is indicated only in the presence of persistent abnormal cell count and protein in the spinal fluid or of a persistent rise in serologic titer. The following are examples of normal and abnormal titers in treated late syphilis. Intervals between tests may be anywhere from 30 to 90 days.

Normal		Abnormal	
Test No.	Titer	Test No.	Titer
1	1:16	1	1:8
2	1:8	2	1:16
3	[1] 1:16	3	[2] 1:32
4	1:8	4	1:64

[1] Differences of one tube in either direction are negligible.
[2] Differences of two tubes or more are considered significant.

Penicillin Sensitivity—Allergic and Anaphylactic Reaction

Severe reactions to penicillin are being reported. For this reason, it is important to get a history of previous allergic reactions to penicillin, or for that matter, of any allergy.

Penicillin should never be administered to anyone who has had a previous reaction to it in any form. Where there is a history of any other serious allergy, penicillin should be administered only with the greatest caution.

In any case, penicillin should never be administered intramuscularly unless the patient may be observed for from 15 minutes to a half hour at minimum.

Some clinicians include routinely injectable antihistamine in each penicillin injection by putting 100 mgm. of antihistamine in each 10 cc. vial of penicillin to be used.

Corticosteroids given routinely along with penicillin may prevent allergic reactions. Early reports indicate good results with this procedure.

Serious anaphylactic reactions and deaths have occurred following the use of penicillin. Although such reactions are extremely rare, emergency measures should be immediately available whenever penicillin is administered.

Anaphylactic reactions may be anticipated by such prodromal symptoms as vertigo, nausea, flushing, itching, or even abdominal pain. The presence of any of these should warrant the administration of two or three inhalations from an adrenalin medihaler. If bronchial spasm or laryngeal edema are not immediately relieved, or if the reaction appears particularly significant at its outset, intravenous adrenalin should be administered, slowly, and with frequent checking of blood pressure.

If indicated, an airtube might be inserted in the trachea; and there are times when a respirator is most useful. Rate should be kept at from 10 to 20 per minute. Where the emergency warrants, an emergency tracheotomy should be performed.

In addition to adrenalin and the foregoing measures, the following medications have also been found helpful:

500 mgm. aminophyllin intravenously,

50 mgm. benadryl hydrochloride intravenously,

800,000 units neutrapen (penicillinase) intravenously.

Should the patient go into shock, his systolic blood pressure falling below 100 mm. of mercury, 500 ml. of 10% glucose in normal saline may be administered intravenously, and 20 mgm. (in 1 ml. ampule) of a vasopressor such as l-norepinephrine may be introduced intravenously at a rate sufficient to maintain adequate blood pressure levels.

Another drug which may be useful in severe shock is Solucortef. Administer 100 mgm. slowly intravenously, either by itself or mixed with glucose in normal saline.

(See Antibiotics, page 12.)

The Herxheimer Reaction

The Jarisch-Herxheimer reaction is presumably caused by the rapid killing of many treponemes. It consists of a transient fever that may or may not be associated with a temporary exacerbation of syphilitic lesions. In a few cases, the latter alone has been observed. The reaction, as a rule, occurs within 12 hours following the first dose of a potent treponemicidal agent. Delayed reactions occurring days or even weeks following the onset of anti-syphilitic therapy have been reported, but it is doubtful whether such reports represent true Herxheimer reactions. The duration of a genuine Herxheimer reaction is usually only a few hours, and rarely more than 24 hours. The reaction is common following the onset of treatment of early syphilis, but it is frequently unnoted by the patient. Following treatment of late syphilis, Herxheimer reactions are rarely noted except in general paresis where abundant treponemes may be present in the cerebral cortex. In some paretics the reaction may cause convulsions or increased agitation requiring restraints or sedatives, but this is not cause for stopping the treatment.

In the pre-penicillin era, serious accidents following arsenical therapy of cardiovascular syphilis were attributed to Herxheimer reactions and the reaction was much feared. Few, if any, authentic Herxheimer reactions following penicillin therapy of cardiovascular syphilis have been noted. It is now generally agreed by most authorities in America that it is safe and advisable to begin treatment of cardiovascular syphilis with the full recommended dose of penicillin, or other effective antibiotics.

APPENDIX

The Lesions of Syphilis

The more common lesions of syphilis are presented on the following pages as an aid to diagnosis. The more devastating lesions of late syphilis, although still occurring, are lacking in these illustrations because it is believed that the average physician will seldom see much severe syphilitic destruction again.

This brings forth a word of caution. Because of widespread use of antibiotics, and perhaps for other reasons as well, the physician should be cautioned that the "typical" syphilitic lesion is not the same as the "classic" lesion. In fact, in view of observations of recent years, it would be difficult to describe a "typical" lesion of syphilis. Those lesions shown here which do not fit the "classical" description are not necessarily atypical.

Where lesions are found which resemble these pictures, they may be highly suggestive of syphilis. But no suspicious lesion of any kind should be ruled out until syphilis itself is ruled out by serology and darkfield.

The following lesions are shown, the numbers of the descriptions corresponding to the numbers of the plates:

Primary Syphilis

Plate
Number
1. Early stage of a darkfield positive chancre on the prepuce.
2. Darkfield positive chancre of the skin of the penis.
3. Darkfield positive chancre on the corona of the glans penis.
4. Darkfield positive chancre of labium majus.
5. Darkfield positive extragenital chancre of the finger.

6. Darkfield positive extragenital chancre of the tongue with typical induration and clean erosive base.

7. Darkfield positive extragenital typical chancre of anterior cheek with satellite submandibular bubo.

8. Darkfield positive extragenital chancre of the upper lip with slight induration, redness, and crusting simulating herpes simplex. Note satellite left submandibular lymph node. These enlarged nodes are firm in consistency and usually painless.

Secondary Syphilis

9. Old pigmented maculopapular syphilid of palms.

10. Palmar syphilid, maculopapular with scaling.

11. Papular syphilid of palms and soles.

12. Maculopapular syphilid of palms.

13. Generalized maculopapular rash with some scaling.

14. Generalized macular rash. This is the most common rash of infectious syphilis. Without good lighting, this could be missed, particularly on the pigmented skin. Cardiolipin antigen (reagin) serology is *always* reactive in secondary syphilis.

15. Annular papular syphilid of face. Darkfield examination of raised border of this type of lesion is usually positive.

16. Generalized papular rash. Darkfield examination of suspect rashes should always be done to confirm diagnosis immediately.

17. Few scattered maculopapular syphilids of palms.

18. Split papules of both commissures.

19. Syphilitic alopecia. Note the "moth eaten" appearance with numerous small areas not completely devoid of hair.

20. Mucous patches of the tongue. Note confluence of lesions, circinate borders and pale grayish membrane. These lesions are highly infectious.

21. Early mucous patches of tongue.

22. Mucous patch on the cervix—also probable site of primary chancre.

23. Small hypertrophic papule (condyloma latum) on right labium minus. Such lesions can be missed unless examination is careful and thorough.

24. Mucous patch of palate. Also note early annular syphilids at lateral margins of nose.

25. Solitary annular syphilid in a young child.
26. Condylomata lata of the male genitalia (scrotum) and adjacent thighs.
27. Condylomata lata of the female genitalia and perianal area. These moist hypertrophic lesions are chronic and highly infectious.
28. Same as 27.
29. Genital and perianal condylomata lata.
30. Hypertrophic moist papules (condylomata lata) in the male perianal area.

Early Congenital Syphilis

31. Snuffles in a syphilitic infant. Also note the split papule on the left emphasizing the infectious stage that some newborn congenitals represent.
32. Annular syphilid in an infant.
33. Eroded perianal maculopapular skin lesions in the newborn illustrating the highly infectious nature of some congenital cases.

Late Congenital Syphilis

34. Interstitial keratitis—an early case showing slight ciliary congestion and small infiltrative deposits at the periphery of the cornea—smarting, discomfort to light, and lacrimation are present.
35. Interstitial keratitis—an advanced case—without adequate therapy, permanent damage to the cornea or iris may be the result.
36. Rhagades (scars) produced by infiltrative syphilids about the mouth and chin in early life.
37. Typical Hutchinson's teeth. The upper central incisors show the peg-shape (pumpkin-seed) central notching, and wide-spacing that make such second dentition (about 6 years and older) diagnostic for congenital syphilis. Unerupted Hutchinson incisors may be identified by dental X-ray at earlier age.
38. Mulberry molar—the first molar of the second dentition (6-year molar) shows a shoulder of enamel bulging around the crown and small defective cusps. These teeth are very much subject to early decay.
39. Saber shins demonstrating the anterior bowing of the tibiae. This is also accompanied by fusiform thickening. Ossifying periostitis in the early months of life or later in the tardive case will produce such bone changes.
40. Clutton's joints—painless bilateral hydrarthrosis of the knees; other joints may be involved—this responds readily to penicillin treatment.

Late Syphilis

41. Solitary ulcerative gumma of the hand. Such lesions can be confused with carbuncles and other non syphilitic lesions.
42. Nodulo-ulcerative late syphilide. The arciform lesions are characteristic.
43. Neurosyphilis—tabes dorsalis—Charcot knee joint illustrating gross destruction.

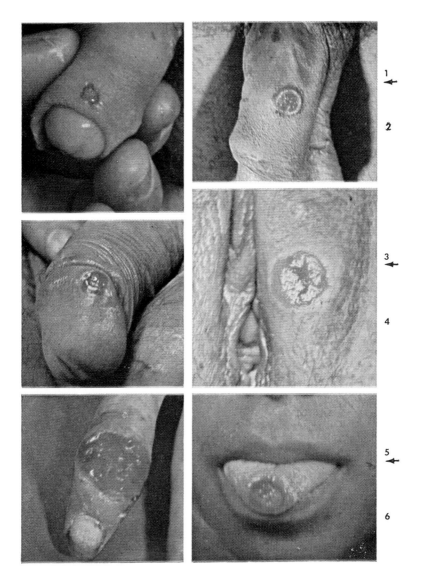

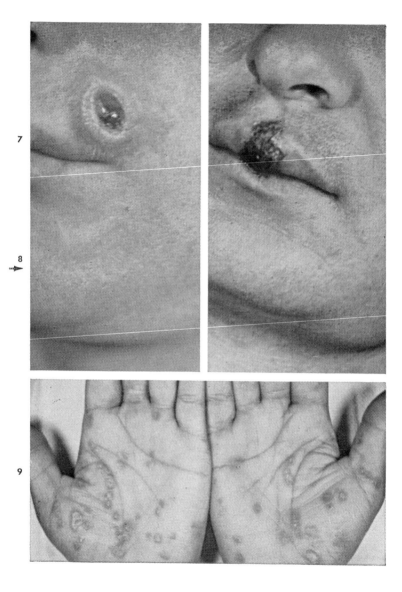

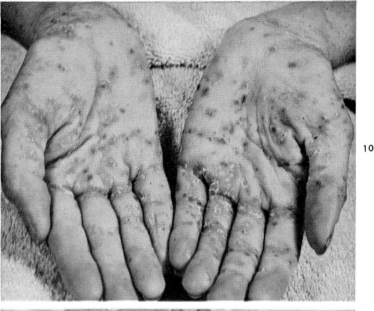

10

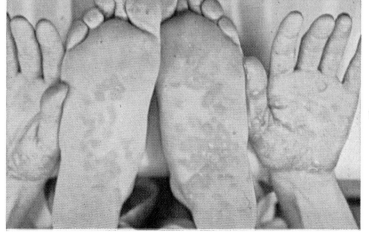

11

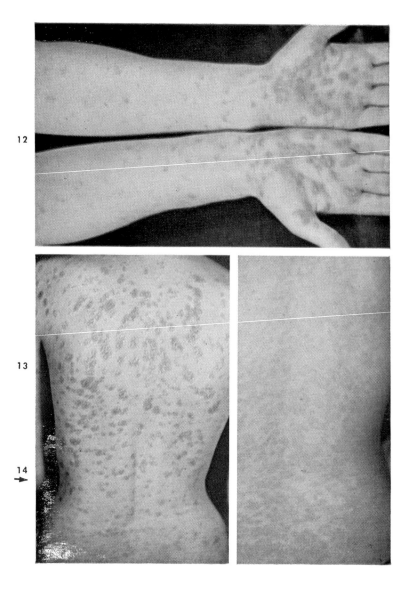

12

13

14 →

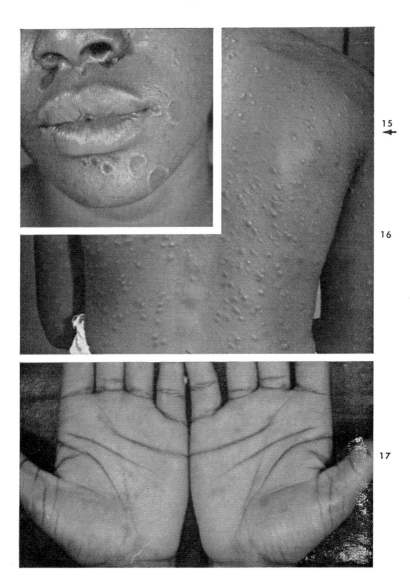

15

16

17

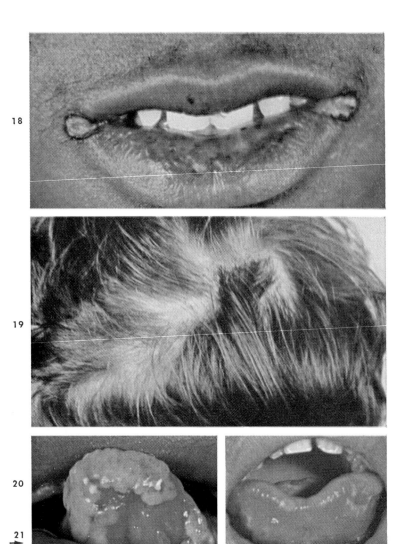

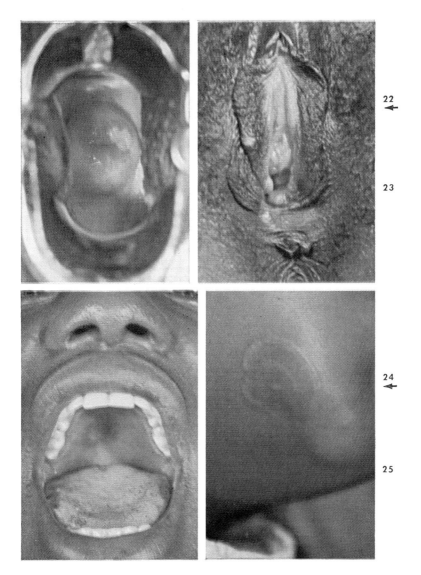

22

23

24

25

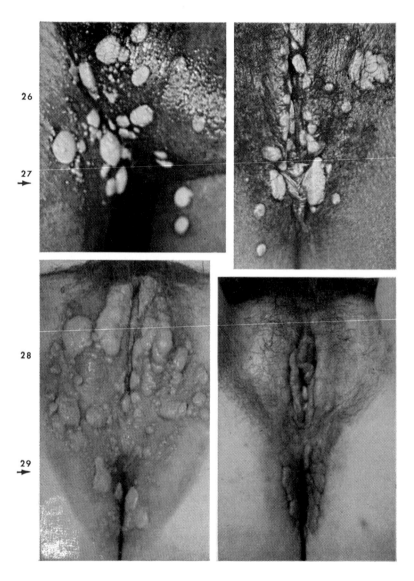

26

27 →

28

29 →

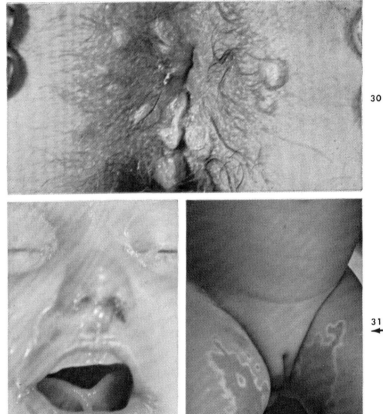

30

31 ←

32

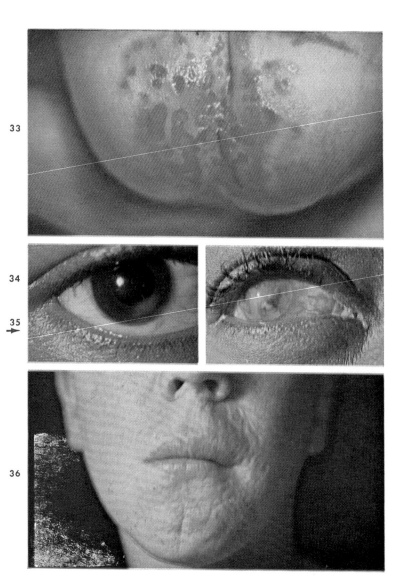

33

34

35

36

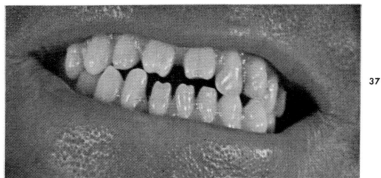

37

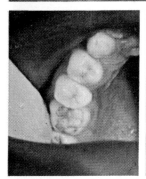

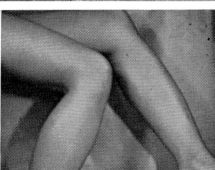

38

39

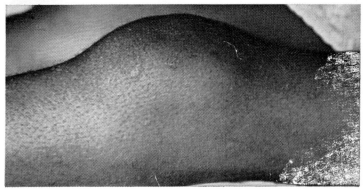

40

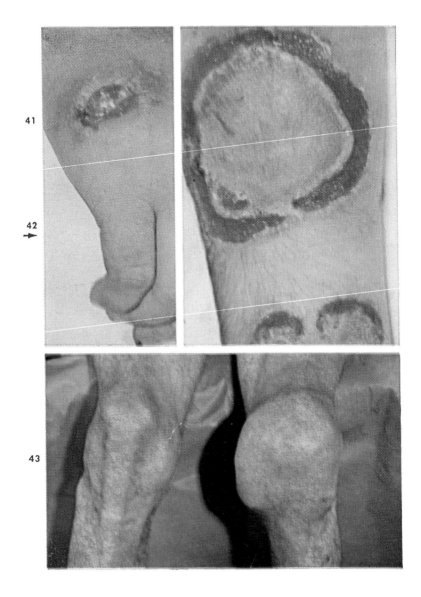

41

42 →

43

An Annotated Bibliography

1. Bulletin of the World Health Organization, 14(2): 1–165, 1956.

    The entire issue is devoted to the laboratory aspects of the treponematosis control program, and includes 24 pages of references grouped under pertinent subject headings. Eight individual articles are represented under the following titles: Serology of treponematoses: Recent developments (Rein and Reyn); Present status of serological tests for syphilis (Harris and Olansky); Biologically false positive reactions to serologic tests for syphilis (Kostant); Modern diagnosis of syphilis (Olansky and Price); Treponema pallidum immobilization test (Nielson and Reyn); Treponema pallidum agglutination tests (Magnuson and McLeod); La Reaction d'adherence—disparations (Daguet); Transmission of blood and serum samples (Price).

2. Hahn, R. D., and others: Penicillin treatment of asymptomatic central nervous system syphilis. I. Probability of progression to symptomatic neurosyphilis. A.M.A. Arch. Dermat., 74(4): 355–366, Oct. 1956.

3. Hahn, R. D., and others: Penicillin treatment of asymptomatic central nervous system syphilis. II. Results of therapy as measured by laboratory findings. A.M.A. Arch. Dermat., 74(4): 367–377, Oct. 1956.

    Pretreatment and posttreatment status of the group of patients referred to in item 6 are discussed on the basis of the blood and spinal fluid examination results, in an effort to evaluate the effectiveness of penicillin therapy.

4. Hahn, R. D., and others: Penicillin treatment of general paresis (Dementia paralytica), Results of treatment in 1,086 patients, the majority of whom were followed for more than 5 years. A.M.A. Arch. Neurol. & Psychiat., 81(5): 557–590, May 1959.

    This is a cooperative study reviewing the clinical, spinal fluid and serologic findings among a group of 1,086 general paretic (dementia paralytica) patients. The group consisted of patients from eight different hospitals who had been treated with penicillin with or without fever therapy. These findings furnished much of the information on which are based current practices in the management of general paresis.

5. Magnuson, H. J.; Thomas, E. V.; Olansky, S.; Kaplan, Bernard I.; Demello, L.; Cutler, J. C.: Inoculation syphilis in human volunteers. Medicine, 35(2): 33–82, Feb. 1956.

   The article discusses a study in which 62 human volunteers at Sing Sing Prison, Ossining, N. Y., were inoculated with virulent Treponema pallidum. Included, also, is a summary of previously reported studies most pertinent to the subject.

6. Moore, J. E.: Seroresistance (Wassermann Fastness): A discussion for the patients. Am. J. Syph., 30(2): 125, Mar. 1946.

   The author discusses, in conversation form between physician and patient, the problems of seroresistance in late (especially latent) syphilis. This is based on an imaginary case and is presented in this form so that reprints might be given to patients.

7. Olansky, S.; and Garson, W.: The treatment of syphilis with antibiotics other than penicillin. A.M.A. Arch. Dermat., 77(6): 648–650, June 1958.

   The authors review pertinent literature, and comment on the clinical effectiveness of some of the various antibiotics currently available to physicians for the treatment of syphilis with an agent other than penicillin. Nineteen references are listed.

8. Stereoscopic Manual of Venereal Disease. Sawyer View-Master, Portland, Oreg., 1955, pp. 1–34.

   In full color, three dimensional photography, this manual presents 98 characteristic clinical manifestations of all the venereal diseases, and of other diseases encountered in differential diagnosis. The illustrations are mounted on 14 View-Master reels. Accompanying text describes each view. Recommended for physicians and students.

9. Stokes, J. A.; Beerman, H.; Ingraham, N. R., Jr.: Modern clinical syphilology. 3d ed. Philadelphia, Saunders, 1945, pp. 1–1332.

   Although some of the material on treatment is outdated, this book, revised last in 1944, remains the most exhaustive single source on all aspects of syphilology and differential diagnosis. Included are 911 illustrations and text figures.

10. Thomas, E. W.: Syphilis: Its course and management. New York, Macmillan, 1949, pp. 1–317.

    An authoritative, concise review of the status of syphilis management in 1949, following 5 years of antibiotic therapy. Written for the general practitioner and the student, it stressed primarily immunology of the disease, the course of untreated syphilis, interpretation of laboratory procedures in diagnosis, and treatment (based primarily on the author's experiences at Bellevue Hospital, New York City).

11. U.S. Department of Health, Education, and Welfare, Public Health Service; Rosahn, P. D.: Autopsy Studies in Syphilis. Public Health Service Pub. No. 433, Washington, D.C., U.S. Government Printing Office, 1955, pp. 1–67.

The monograph presents a summary of a survey of 5,300 autopsies in the Department of Pathology, Yale University School of Medicine, since 1917. Additional information from pertinent literature is included.

12. U.S. Department of Health, Education, and Welfare, Public Health Service: Serology Evaluation and Research Assembly, 1956–1957. Public Health Service Pub. No. 650, Washington, D.C., U.S. Government Printing Office.

This official report of an evaluation of serologic tests for syphilis, conducted by the Public Health Service through the cooperation of 15 laboratories, includes a comparative analysis of the performance of 12 Treponema pallidum, 7 Reiter treponeme, and 18 nontreponemal antigen techniques in testing. A total of 1,298 specimens represented 10 syphilitic and nonsyphilitic categories.

13. U.S. Department of Health, Education, and Welfare, Public Health Service: Laboratory Procedures for Modern Syphilis Serology. Communicable Disease Center, Atlanta, Ga., July 1961.

New modifications of technical serologic procedures as recommended by test-author serologists are incorporated in this publication. Procedures, in complete detail, are given for the following: (1) VDRL Slide Flocculation Tests with Serum, (2) VDRL Slide Flocculation Tests with Spinal Fluid, (3) Rapid Plasma Reagin Test, (4) Unheated Serum Reagin Test, (5) Reiter Protein Antigen Test (Kolmer), (6) Fluorescent Treponemal Antibody Test (FTA). These represent the most widely used of the older procedures and the newer tests of current interest.

A Note on Source Material

MANY kinds of materials are available to professional persons interested in the pursuit of further knowledge about syphilis and the other venereal diseases. One of the principal sources of such materials is the Venereal Disease Program of the Communicable Disease Center, Public Health Service, Department of Health, Education, and Welfare, which maintains research laboratories, statistical services, and informational and educational services, along with a mobile field staff of trained venereal disease epidemiologists.

Inquiries may be addressed to Chief, Venereal Disease Branch, Communicable Disease Center, Atlanta, Ga.

Mailing lists. Two mailing lists are maintained, one for professional and public health persons only, the other for persons interested in venereal disease information and education. The first list is for the periodic mailing of "Current Literature on Venereal Disease," a collection of abstracts of current venereal disease literature from more than 800 journals of many languages. These collections are distributed three or four times a year and indexed annually. The second list, called the "Educational Distribution List," aims to keep interested persons informed as to the latest venereal disease informational and educational materials as they become available. In many cases, sample copies are mailed or offered. Names are added to either or both of these lists only on specific request.

Audio visuals. Films, filmographs, slides, pictures, manuals, and reprints are loaned or distributed on request. Scientific and public health exhibits are offered to appropriate gatherings.

Bibliographic research. On request, special bibliographies are prepared on related special subjects from files which go back to 1920. Technical inquiries relating to the latest findings of research studies constantly in progress in the field of diagnosis and management receive prompt and serious attention.

○